THE HONEST GLP-1 GUIDE

What Most People Aren’t Told About GLP-1 Therapy, Muscle Loss, Plateaus, and Long-Term Metabolic Health

Sylvalene Alozie, DNP, APRN, FNP-C

Contents

THE HONEST GLP-1 GUIDE What Most People Aren’t Told About GLP-1 Therapy, Muscle Loss, Plateaus, and Long-Term Metabolic Health Sylvalene Alozie, DNP, APRN, FNP-C

Printed in the United States of America

Medical Disclaimer

The content in this book is provided for educational purposes only and is not intended to replace individualized medical care. GLP-1, or glucagon-like peptide-1 medications and other weight-loss therapies should only be initiated and managed under the supervision of a qualified healthcare professional.

Individual outcomes vary. No guarantees of specific results are made or implied.

If you believe you may have a medical emergency, contact emergency services immediately.

DEDICATION

For those seeking clarity where noise has replaced understanding — and for the clinicians who continue to lead with balance, integrity, and thoughtful care.

Contents

How to Use This Book

GLP-1 therapy is often discussed in fragments — a side effect here, a dosing schedule there, a before-and-after story without context. This guide was written differently. It is structured to move from physiology to psychology to long-term strategy so readers can understand not only what GLP-1 therapy does, but how to think about it within the larger framework of metabolic health.

"As a clinician working within metabolic medicine, my goal is not to simplify GLP-1 therapy into trends, but to place it within a clear framework of physiology, muscle preservation, and long-term metabolic care."

You do not need to read this book in a single sitting. Some readers will move sequentially from the Introduction through the final chapters. Others may choose to focus on specific areas depending on where they are in their journey.

If you are considering starting GLP-1 therapy: Begin with Chapters 1–4 to understand metabolic context, appetite signaling, and what is actually being treated.

If you are currently using GLP-1 therapy: Focus on Chapters 5–8 and Chapter 12, which address rapid weight loss, muscle preservation, monitoring, and building metabolic infrastructure.

If you are thinking about long-term planning or discontinuation: Chapters 10–14 provide perspective on appropriate use, maintenance models, and expectations over time.

Throughout the book, you will see a brief section titled Clinician Bottom Line at the end of many chapters. These summaries highlight the central clinical takeaway — the perspective I want readers to remember long after the details fade.

This guide is not meant to replace individualized medical care. Instead, it is designed to help you enter conversations with greater clarity, stronger expectations, and a deeper understanding of how GLP-1 therapy fits within long-term metabolic health.

You are encouraged to read at your own pace, revisit sections as needed, and focus less on speed and more on understanding. Sustainable outcomes are rarely built on urgency. They are built on clarity, structure, and consistency.

Author's Note

GLP-1 medications entered public conversation rapidly. With rapid visibility comes simplification. In clinical practice, I see the same pattern repeatedly: patients arrive with strong opinions and weak context—either expecting a miracle or fearing a shortcut. Neither extreme supports good outcomes.

This book was written to restore clinical balance. GLP-1 therapy can be highly effective, but effectiveness is not the same as durability. The medication can quiet appetite and improve metabolic markers while it is active. What determines long-term results is what gets built around it—muscle preservation, nutritional structure, realistic expectations, and ongoing oversight.

My position is straightforward: GLP-1 is a tool, not a strategy. Used thoughtfully, it can change trajectories. Used without structure, it often produces short-term loss followed by long-term frustration.

This guide offers clarity without exaggeration—grounded in physiology, behavior, and the realities clinicians see after the initial excitement fades.

– Sylvalene Alozie, DNP, APRN, FNP-C

A clinician's position on GLP-1 therapy: The medication can reduce biological resistance to change – but long-term success depends on muscle preservation, metabolic structure, and realistic expectations.

Clinical Context The perspective in this book reflects active clinical experience in virtual metabolic health management. In practice, the most common problem is not the medication. It is the model surrounding it: inadequate protein intake, minimal resistance training, unrealistic expectations, and weak follow-up.

GLP-1 therapy should always be individualized, medically supervised, and aligned with a long-term metabolic plan. This book is designed to strengthen informed conversations and decision-making. It does not replace clinical evaluation, diagnosis, or individualized medical care.

Introduction - The Injection Everyone Is Talking About

There are rare moments in medicine when a treatment crosses into mainstream culture. GLP-1 medications did. They moved from endocrinology clinics into celebrity interviews, social media threads, telehealth ads, and everyday conversation. Suddenly, weight loss was no longer framed only as willpower, calorie counting, or gym consistency. It became about injections. About biology. About something that finally seemed to work.

For many people, it does.

But when results are fast, visible, and public, the conversation becomes noisy. Physiology gets replaced by before-and-after photos. Expectations rise faster than understanding. And the same pattern appears repeatedly: people start therapy believing they are treating hunger alone—when they are actually entering a system that influences appetite signaling, reward pathways, gastric emptying, insulin dynamics, body composition, and long-term metabolic adaptation.

As a clinician, I have watched the public narrative swing between two extremes: miracle cure or moral shortcut. Neither is clinically accurate. GLP-1 medications are not magic. They are not a failure of discipline. They are not a personality change in a syringe.

They are tools—powerful tools.

And here is the honest part that many people learn too late: a tool can create change, but it cannot create structure. The medication can quiet appetite. It cannot preserve muscle for you. It cannot build strength. It cannot stabilize sleep. It cannot correct chronic stress physiology. It cannot teach nutrition. And it cannot carry the full weight of maintenance once the early momentum slows—which it almost always does.

This guide exists for one purpose: clarity. Not fear. Not hype. Not marketing.

Inside these pages, we will examine what GLP-1 therapy actually does in the brain and body, why results vary, why plateaus are normal, and why muscle preservation is the difference between "smaller" and "metabolically stronger." We will also discuss safety, monitoring, and what discontinuation realistically looks like—because long-term success depends on planning, not optimism.

You deserve realistic expectations. You deserve clinically grounded guidance. And you deserve a framework that treats weight regulation as metabolic care—not a social media storyline.

“GLP-1 therapy is not the strategy itself; it is a metabolic lever – and long-term outcomes depend on what is built while that lever is in motion.”

GLP-1 therapy can be life-changing. But it is not the entire story. This book explains the rest.

“GLP-1 therapy may quiet the signal of hunger, but what ultimately determines the outcome is the structure built while the signal is quiet.”

– Sylvalene Alozie, DNP, APRN, FNP-C

Chapter 1 - Why GLP-1 Exploded

GLP-1 medications did not become mainstream because people suddenly abandoned discipline. They became mainstream because, for the first time in decades, a weight-management medication produced results that were both visible and repeatable—without stimulant dependency and without the high-profile safety failures that undermined earlier drug eras.

For years, weight management lived in a frustrating space between advice and biology.

Eat less. Move more. Try harder.

Many people followed that advice. Some lost weight. Many regained it. Over time, the cycle reinforced a cultural narrative that excess weight reflected character rather than physiology.

Then came medications such as semaglutide and tirzepatide.

These therapies targeted appetite regulation at the neurohormonal level. They influenced insulin response. They slowed gastric emptying. Most notably, they reduced what many patients describe as "food noise"—the persistent cognitive preoccupation with eating, negotiating, craving, and resisting.

For many individuals, the shift felt profound. The internal dialogue changed from:

"Why can't I control this?" to "Why wasn't this explained sooner?"

Scientific advancement alone, however, does not create cultural momentum.

Visibility does.

Celebrity disclosures accelerated awareness. Social media amplified dramatic transformations. Telehealth platforms reduced access barriers. Marketing campaigns simplified complex physiology into digestible slogans. A medication class became a mainstream phenomenon.

And when medical treatments enter popular culture, nuance often disappears.

Results are showcased. Mechanisms are abbreviated. Expectations inflate.

Rarely discussed—yet clinically central—are the realities of:

• Physiologic adaptation • Muscle preservation • Weight-loss variability • Plateau phases • Long-term maintenance

The public narrative became binary: miracle or mistake. Neither is accurate.

GLP-1 medications represent a meaningful advancement in metabolic treatment. They also represent a test of how medical progress is interpreted in the age of virality. Rapid adoption does not eliminate the need for education. Access does not replace understanding. Visible weight loss does not automatically equal metabolic health.

GLP-1 therapy expanded quickly for a simple reason:

It works.

The confusion that followed is equally simple:

Success without context creates distortion.

This book exists to restore that context—so patients pursue outcomes that last, not outcomes that trend.

Clinician Bottom Line GLP-1 therapy can reduce physiologic resistance to change, but it does not replace metabolic structure. The most durable outcomes occur when muscle preservation, nutritional strategy, realistic expectations, and clinical oversight remain central to the process. The goal is not simply rapid weight loss. The goal is long-term metabolic stability.

Chapter 2 - Metabolic Disease: What's Actually Being Treated

Before discussing medication, a more fundamental question must be addressed:

What problem is actually being treated?

GLP-1 therapy is often framed as a weight-loss solution. But weight is a visible outcome—not the underlying pathology. In clinical practice, the focus is rarely the number on the scale alone. The deeper issue is metabolic regulation: how the body manages energy, hunger signaling, insulin dynamics, and adaptation over time.

For many individuals, excess weight reflects metabolic dysregulation rather than simple caloric imbalance. Understanding that distinction changes not only treatment decisions, but expectations.

Obesity as a Chronic Disease

Obesity is increasingly recognized as a chronic, relapsing, multifactorial disease. It is influenced by:

• Neurohormonal signaling • Genetic predisposition • Environmental exposure • Behavioral patterns • Sleep architecture • Stress physiology • Medication effects

Reducing this condition to "eat less and move more" ignores the regulatory systems governing body weight. Appetite, satiety, and energy expenditure are not static variables controlled solely by intention. They are biologically defended processes.

This does not remove personal responsibility. It reframes the environment in which that responsibility operates.

The Set Point and the Body's Defense System

The human body defends weight.

Many researchers describe this as a "set point"—a biologically regulated range that the body attempts to maintain through adjustments in hunger, satiety, and energy expenditure. Others use the term "settling point," reflecting a dynamic interaction between biology and environment. Regardless of terminology, the principle remains consistent:

When weight decreases significantly, the body adapts.

Common physiologic responses include:

• Increased hunger signaling • Reduced satiety signaling • Lower resting metabolic rate • Heightened sensitivity to food reward

These responses are not evidence of weak willpower. They are evolutionary protections designed to prevent starvation.

This is one reason weight regain after traditional dieting is so common. The body is not resisting change out of defiance. It is defending equilibrium.

Visceral vs. Subcutaneous Fat

Not all adipose tissue behaves the same.

Subcutaneous fat lies beneath the skin. Visceral fat surrounds internal organs.

Visceral adipose tissue is metabolically active and associated with:

• Insulin resistance • Inflammatory signaling • Cardiovascular risk • Hepatic fat accumulation

Two individuals with similar body weight may have very different metabolic profiles depending on fat distribution. This is why weight alone does not fully define health status.

GLP-1 therapy often reduces visceral adiposity, which helps explain improvements in cardiometabolic markers beyond scale reduction.

Insulin Resistance and Energy Partitioning

Insulin is a storage hormone. In metabolically stable states, it allows glucose to enter cells efficiently. In insulin resistance:

• Cells respond less effectively to insulin • Circulating insulin levels may rise • Fat storage becomes easier • Fat mobilization becomes more difficult • Energy stability declines

The result is often misunderstood as lack of discipline. Clinically, it reflects signaling distortion.

GLP-1 therapy influences insulin dynamics, but insulin resistance typically develops over years. No medication erases long-standing physiology overnight. It modulates the system while active.

Weight Cycling and Metabolic Adaptation

Repeated cycles of aggressive dieting followed by regain—often called weight cycling—can amplify metabolic resistance.

Each cycle may contribute to:

• Lean mass loss • Reduced resting metabolic rate • Heightened hunger signaling • Greater biologic defense against further loss

Over time, patients often say, "It's harder now than it used to be." That perception is frequently physiologic reality.

The body becomes more efficient at conserving energy.

Efficiency is protective. It is not always metabolically helpful.

Adaptive Thermogenesis

As body weight decreases, energy expenditure often drops beyond what would be predicted by body size alone. This phenomenon—adaptive thermogenesis—explains why progress slows even when behaviors remain consistent.

Fewer calories are burned at rest. Movement efficiency improves. The original deficit narrows.

A plateau does not automatically indicate behavioral failure. It often reflects metabolic adaptation.

Understanding this reduces unnecessary dose escalation and frustration.

Why Calorie Math Fails Long Term

Calorie equations assume static systems.

Human physiology is not static.

As weight decreases:

• Hunger signaling increases • Energy expenditure decreases • Hormonal feedback loops shift • Food reward sensitivity may rise

The deficit that produced early loss may no longer produce the same results later. This is not inconsistency—it is recalibration.

Calorie math explains short-term change. It does not guarantee durability.

Reframing the Objective

If excess weight is viewed solely as a behavioral problem, treatment becomes narrow. If it is viewed as a chronic metabolic condition, the objective expands.

The goal becomes restoring metabolic stability.

Weight reduction becomes one marker among many, alongside:

• Improved insulin sensitivity • Reduced visceral adiposity • Preserved lean mass • Stable energy regulation • Lower inflammatory burden • Long-term cardiometabolic resilience

GLP-1 therapy may support these outcomes. It is not the outcome itself.

The Honest Clinical Context

Patients often ask, "Does this medication fix metabolism?"

The most accurate answer is:

It supports metabolic regulation while active.

Chronic conditions require chronic strategy. Medication may be part of that strategy. Structure must always be.

Clinician Bottom Line GLP-1 therapy can reduce physiologic resistance to change, but it does not replace metabolic structure. The most durable outcomes occur when muscle preservation, nutritional strategy, realistic expectations, and clinical oversight remain central to the process. The goal is not simply rapid weight loss. The goal is long-term metabolic stability.

Chapter 3 - Appetite, Reward, and Food Noise

Hunger is not a character flaw. It is a neurobiological signal.

To understand why GLP-1 therapy feels different from traditional dieting, it is necessary to distinguish between homeostatic hunger and reward-driven eating.

They are not identical systems. They overlap — but they are regulated differently.

Understanding this distinction changes how weight regulation is interpreted.

Homeostatic Hunger: Survival Signaling

Homeostatic hunger is driven by energy need.

When the body requires fuel, hormonal signals coordinate appetite regulation:

Ghrelin rises to stimulate hunger

Leptin communicates energy sufficiency

Insulin participates in satiety signaling

The hypothalamus integrates metabolic input

This system evolved for survival.

When energy stores decline, hunger increases. When energy stores are replenished, satiety follows.

In metabolically stable individuals, this system operates within predictable boundaries.

In individuals with chronic metabolic dysregulation, signaling may become amplified or distorted:

Hunger may feel more urgent

Satiety may feel delayed

Cravings may feel persistent

The experience becomes less predictable — and more effortful.

This is not weakness. It is signaling dysregulation.

Hedonic Eating: The Reward Circuit

Separate from survival-driven hunger is reward-driven eating.

This system involves dopaminergic signaling within:

The ventral tegmental area

The nucleus accumbens

The prefrontal cortex

These regions regulate motivation, anticipation, and reinforcement.

Highly palatable foods — particularly those combining sugar, fat, and salt — stimulate dopamine release independent of caloric necessity.

This produces reinforcement.

Repeated exposure strengthens habit loops:

Cue Anticipation Consumption Reward Reinforcement

Over time, anticipation itself becomes rewarding.

This anticipatory activation is often what patients describe as:

“Food noise.”

Not hunger.

Preoccupation.

Mental negotiation.

Persistent cognitive background activity centered on food.

The Modern Food Environment

The current food environment intensifies reward circuitry activation.

Ultra-processed foods are engineered for hyper-palatability. They are rapidly absorbed, highly stimulating, and widely accessible.

This creates a mismatch between ancient survival circuitry and modern availability.

The brain interprets these stimuli as high-value resources.

Repeated exposure reinforces:

Habit loops

Emotional association

Environmental cue conditioning

The result is not lack of discipline.

It is predictable neuroadaptation.

What GLP-1 Therapy Modulates

GLP-1 receptor activation influences both homeostatic and reward pathways.

Clinically, many individuals report:

Reduced hunger intensity

Earlier satiety

Reduced impulsivity around food

Decreased cognitive preoccupation

The internal volume decreases.

The negotiation quiets.

For individuals accustomed to persistent effort, this shift can feel transformative.

It is not simply appetite suppression.

It is signaling modulation.

The medication dampens both hunger intensity and reward salience.

Dopamine and Reinforcement Reset

Chronic exposure to hyper-palatable foods can alter dopamine sensitivity.

Over time:

Higher stimulation is required for the same reward

Anticipation becomes exaggerated

Self-regulation becomes more effortful

GLP-1 therapy appears to reduce reward sensitivity to highly palatable foods.

Patients frequently report: “I don’t think about food the same way.”

This is not a personality change.

It is altered reinforcement signaling.

However, modulation is not permanent rewiring.

When medication is discontinued, reward sensitivity may normalize.

Structure determines whether previous patterns reemerge.

Behavioral Exposure

When food noise decreases, something unexpected can occur.

Silence exposes structure.

For some individuals, reduced preoccupation creates relief and cognitive space.

For others, it reveals how much food previously served as:

Stress regulation

Emotional buffering

Distraction

Ritual

The medication quiets appetite.

It does not replace coping systems.

This is not medication failure.

It is behavioral exposure.

Identity and Eating

Food is rarely just fuel.

It is culture. It is memory. It is social bonding. It is comfort.

When appetite decreases pharmacologically, emotional associations do not automatically recalibrate.

This can create tension:

"I'm not hungry – but I still want to eat."

Recognizing the difference between physiologic hunger and conditioned desire is foundational.

GLP-1 therapy makes the distinction observable.

It does not eliminate the need for awareness.

The Opportunity Window

The greatest clinical value of GLP-1 therapy may not be rapid weight reduction.

It may be the creation of an opportunity window.

During this period:

Appetite resistance is reduced

Cognitive load decreases

Behavioral change requires less negotiation

If used intentionally, this window allows:

Nutritional structure to stabilize

Protein prioritization to become routine

Stress responses to be addressed

Identity to recalibrate

If used passively, it becomes temporary suppression.

Interruption is not reconstruction.

Reconstruction requires structure.

Clinician Bottom Line GLP-1 therapy can reduce physiologic resistance to change, but it does not replace metabolic structure. The most durable outcomes occur when muscle preservation, nutritional strategy, realistic expectations, and clinical oversight remain central to the process. The goal is not simply rapid weight loss. The goal is long-term metabolic stability.

Chapter 4 - Beyond Appetite: Insulin, Inflammation, and Metabolic Signaling

Appetite reduction is the most visible effect of GLP-1 therapy. It is not the only effect.

Weight management is not governed solely by hunger. It is influenced by hormonal signaling, glucose regulation, inflammatory pathways, and energy partitioning. Understanding these systems clarifies why GLP-1 medications can affect more than body weight.

Insulin and Energy Storage Insulin is a storage hormone. When functioning appropriately, it helps move glucose into cells for energy use or storage. When signaling becomes dysregulated, energy handling shifts.

In insulin resistance:

Cells respond less efficiently to insulin

Circulating insulin levels may rise

Fat storage becomes easier

Fat mobilization becomes more difficult

Energy levels may fluctuate

The result can include hunger variability, energy instability, and gradual weight gain.

GLP-1 therapies influence insulin secretion in a glucose-dependent manner. Insulin release is enhanced when glucose is elevated, rather than indiscriminately. This supports improved glycemic control and generally reduces hypoglycemia risk in most individuals (particularly in the absence of other glucose-lowering agents). Insulin regulation, however, is only one component of metabolic balance.

Glucose Variability and Appetite Glucose fluctuations can influence hunger perception. Rapid spikes followed by rapid declines may contribute to increased appetite, cravings, and fatigue.

Stabilizing postprandial glucose often reduces these oscillations. GLP-1 medications slow gastric emptying and modulate insulin response, which can contribute to smoother glycemic patterns. For some individuals, improved glucose stability reduces urgency around eating. This is not simply “less hunger.” It is more stable signaling.

Inflammation and Metabolic Stress Chronic low-grade inflammation is frequently associated with excess adiposity and insulin resistance. Adipose tissue is metabolically active and releases signaling molecules that influence inflammatory pathways.

Reducing adipose mass can:

Lower inflammatory burden

Improve vascular function

Enhance insulin sensitivity

Reduce cardiometabolic risk markers

GLP-1 therapy may contribute indirectly through weight reduction and improved metabolic signaling. However, inflammation is also influenced by sleep, stress, physical activity, and nutritional quality. Medication can modulate one axis. Systemic resilience typically requires multiple.

Energy Partitioning Not all weight loss is metabolically equal.

Energy partitioning refers to how the body allocates energy—toward fat storage, muscle maintenance, or expenditure. Without adequate protein intake and resistance training, caloric reduction may result in disproportionate lean mass loss. With structural reinforcement, the body is more likely to preserve muscle while reducing adipose tissue.

GLP-1 therapy influences intake. It does not determine partitioning. Behavior and structure do.

Cardiometabolic Markers Beyond weight, clinicians often track:

Hemoglobin A1c

Fasting glucose

Fasting insulin (when appropriate)

Lipid profiles

Blood pressure

Inflammatory markers (selectively)

GLP-1 therapies have demonstrated improvements across several of these parameters in appropriate populations. These shifts are clinically meaningful and help reframe the conversation from cosmetic reduction to metabolic health. They do not eliminate the need for monitoring or longitudinal assessment.

The System Perspective Metabolic health is not governed by a single hormone. It is an integrated system: appetite signaling, insulin regulation, energy expenditure, muscle mass, sleep architecture, and stress response interact continuously.

GLP-1 therapy influences key regulatory nodes within this system. It does not override the system itself. This distinction protects expectations and supports more stable long-term planning.

Clinician Bottom Line GLP-1 therapy can reduce physiologic resistance to change, but it does not replace metabolic structure. The most durable outcomes occur when muscle preservation, nutritional strategy, realistic expectations, and clinical oversight remain central to the process. The goal is not simply rapid weight loss. The goal is long-term metabolic stability.

Chapter 5 - Behavioral Adaptation During Rapid Weight Loss

Rapid weight loss alters more than physiology. It alters perception.

When body weight changes quickly, external responses often shift before internal identity does. Clothing fits differently. Photographs feel unfamiliar. Comments increase.

For some individuals, this feels empowering. For others, destabilizing.

Few are prepared for that distinction.

Identity Lag

The body can change faster than self-concept.

This creates what may be described as identity lag — a period during which the external image no longer aligns with internal perception.

Individuals may still think of themselves through the lens of their previous weight. Social interactions may feel incongruent. Compliments may feel uncomfortable.

This is not vanity. It is neurological adaptation.

The brain updates more slowly than the scale.

External Validation

Weight loss rarely occurs privately.

Questions emerge: "How much have you lost?" "What are you taking?" "Are you going to stay on it?"

Attention increases. Opinions surface.

External validation can subtly redirect motivation. Health improvements may become secondary to appearance feedback. Progress can begin to feel performative rather than personal.

External validation is unstable.

When motivation shifts outward, durability weakens.

The Performance Mindset

Early progress during GLP-1 therapy often feels decisive.

Five pounds becomes ten. Ten becomes twenty. Momentum builds.

The brain adapts quickly to improvement. What once felt extraordinary becomes expected. The timeline compresses.

Speed becomes conflated with success.

But speed is not durability.

When rapid progress slows — as physiology dictates it will — individuals may interpret adaptation as regression. That misinterpretation fuels unnecessary anxiety.

Emotional Displacement

Food frequently serves multiple roles:

Comfort

Celebration

Stress relief

Distraction

Control

When appetite decreases pharmacologically, these behavioral functions become more visible.

Some individuals experience relief. Others experience exposure.

Without the familiar reinforcement of eating, unresolved stress patterns may surface more clearly.

This is not medication failure. It is behavioral recalibration.

The Risk of All-or-Nothing Thinking

Rapid results can amplify cognitive extremes:

“If this works, I must do it perfectly.” “If progress slows, I am failing.”

All-or-nothing thinking is incompatible with metabolic durability.

Sustainable change is iterative, not absolute.

GLP-1 therapy reduces appetite resistance. It does not eliminate cognitive distortion.

Redefining Progress

The most durable outcomes occur when progress is redefined.

Not solely:

Lower scale weight

Smaller clothing size

But also:

Improved laboratory markers

Preserved strength

Stable energy

Reduced preoccupation with food

Emotional regulation independent of eating

The scale is a data point. It is not identity.

Clinician Bottom Line GLP-1 therapy can reduce physiologic resistance to change, but it does not replace metabolic structure. The most durable outcomes occur when muscle preservation, nutritional strategy, realistic expectations, and clinical oversight remain central to the process. The goal is not simply rapid weight loss. The goal is long-term metabolic stability.

Chapter 6 - The Muscle Loss Nobody Warned You About

When most people talk about GLP-1 therapy, they talk about pounds.

They rarely talk about composition.

The scale measures total mass. It does not distinguish between adipose tissue, skeletal muscle, glycogen, fluid, or bone. When weight decreases rapidly—as it often does during GLP-1 therapy—the body draws energy from multiple sources.

That includes muscle.

This is one of the most important conversations missing from the public narrative. Rapid weight reduction without intentional muscle preservation may create a smaller body that is metabolically weaker.

Weight loss is visible. Muscle loss is quieter. But metabolically, it matters more.

The Scale Is an Incomplete Tool

A standard scale reflects total body weight—not structural change. Early weight loss frequently includes:

• Glycogen depletion • Fluid shifts • Fat mass reduction • Lean mass reduction

The number may drop quickly, but the composition of that drop determines long-term outcome.

Two individuals may lose the same amount of weight and experience entirely different metabolic trajectories depending on how much lean tissue is preserved.

The scale does not reveal that difference.

Lean Mass Is Not Just Muscle — But Muscle Matters Most

In clinical research, "lean mass" includes everything that is not fat: skeletal muscle, organs, connective tissue, and intracellular water. When studies report lean mass loss during weight reduction, skeletal muscle often represents the most clinically relevant component.

Muscle is not cosmetic. It is functional infrastructure.

It supports:

• Insulin sensitivity • Glucose disposal • Resting metabolic expenditure • Physical stability and mobility • Long-term maintenance capacity

Loss of skeletal muscle weakens metabolic resilience—even when total weight improves.

Why Rapid Weight Loss Can Sacrifice Muscle

During significant caloric reduction:

• Protein intake often declines unintentionally • Resistance training may become inconsistent • Fatigue may reduce movement • The body prioritizes efficiency

Without sufficient amino acid intake and mechanical stimulus, muscle protein breakdown may increase. The body is not "failing." It is adapting to perceived energy scarcity.

This is not unique to GLP-1 therapy. It occurs in many rapid weight-loss states. The difference is whether preservation is intentional.

GLP-1 medications reduce appetite. They do not prioritize protein intake. They do not schedule resistance training.

That responsibility remains external to the prescription.

The "Smaller but Weaker" Pattern

Some individuals describe feeling lighter yet less stable or less strong.

Clinically, this may reflect:

• Reduced lean mass • Lower absolute strength • Declining metabolic rate

Weight decreases. Capacity may also decrease.

A smaller body is not automatically a stronger body.

Metabolic reinforcement—not simply reduction—should be the objective.

Energy Partitioning: Where Weight Loss Comes From

Energy partitioning describes how the body allocates energy during weight change—toward fat loss, muscle preservation, or muscle breakdown.

Several factors influence partitioning:

• Adequate protein intake • Resistance training stimulus • Sleep quality • Hormonal environment • Overall nutritional sufficiency

GLP-1 therapy influences intake. Behavior influences partitioning.

When intake decreases without structure, lean tissue becomes vulnerable.

The Metabolic Cost of Muscle Loss

Skeletal muscle contributes meaningfully to resting energy expenditure. When muscle declines:

• Basal metabolic rate may decrease • Glucose regulation becomes less efficient • Maintenance becomes more difficult

This helps explain why aggressive dieting often leads to later regain. The body becomes more energy-efficient.

Efficiency is biologically protective. It is not always metabolically advantageous.

The Visual Illusion

Fat loss and muscle loss can appear similar on the scale—but the physiologic outcomes differ.

Fat loss with preserved muscle:

• Maintains structure • Supports insulin sensitivity • Preserves strength

Fat loss accompanied by muscle loss:

• Reduces metabolic capacity • Weakens resilience • Increases long-term regain risk

The distinction is not aesthetic. It is physiologic.

Measuring Composition

Several tools attempt to estimate body composition:

• DEXA scans • Bioelectrical impedance analysis • Skinfold measurements • Imaging modalities in research settings

No tool is perfect. Each carries limitations. But awareness of composition shifts the conversation from pounds to physiology.

Weight alone does not define progress.

Reframing Success

The objective of GLP-1 therapy should not be weight reduction at any cost.

It should be intelligent loss:

• Fat reduction • Muscle preservation • Stable metabolic function

This requires intention:

• Adequate protein intake—even when hunger is low • Consistent resistance training • Avoiding extreme caloric restriction beyond medication effect • Monitoring energy, strength, and recovery

GLP-1 therapy can create momentum. Structure determines durability.

Clinician Bottom Line GLP-1 therapy can reduce physiologic resistance to change, but it does not replace metabolic structure. The most durable outcomes occur when muscle preservation, nutritional strategy, realistic expectations, and clinical oversight remain central to the process. The goal is not simply rapid weight loss. The goal is long-term metabolic stability.

Chapter 7 - Metabolic Adaptation and the Plateau Phase

Weight loss does not occur in a vacuum.

It occurs within aging physiology.

After the age of 30, skeletal muscle mass begins to decline gradually. This process accelerates with age. Without resistance training and adequate protein intake, the decline compounds.

This matters more than most people realize.

Sarcopenia: The Silent Shift

Sarcopenia refers to the age-related loss of skeletal muscle mass and strength.

It is not dramatic at first. It is incremental.

Muscle tissue influences:

Insulin sensitivity

Glucose disposal

Resting metabolic rate

Balance and fall prevention

Bone density

Physical independence

When muscle declines, metabolic resilience declines with it.

In the context of rapid weight loss, lean mass reduction may compound age-related muscle loss.

This is not cosmetic.

It is physiologic.

Muscle as Metabolic Currency

Muscle is metabolically active tissue.

It functions as a primary site of glucose uptake. After meals, skeletal muscle absorbs circulating glucose under insulin signaling. The more muscle present, the greater the metabolic buffering capacity.

Reduced muscle mass may contribute to:

Worsened insulin sensitivity

Higher postprandial glucose excursions

Reduced resting metabolic rate

Increased fatigue

Weight reduction that sacrifices muscle weakens this buffering system.

The goal is not smaller mass.

It is stronger composition.

Protein Thresholds and Muscle Signaling

Muscle preservation is not automatic.

Muscle protein synthesis requires adequate amino acid availability, particularly leucine — an essential amino acid that triggers muscle-building signaling pathways.

When appetite declines on GLP-1 therapy:

Protein intake may drop unintentionally

Total caloric intake may fall below optimal levels

Meal frequency may decline

If protein intake remains insufficient, muscle protein synthesis decreases.

While individual needs vary, most adults undergoing weight reduction benefit from deliberate protein prioritization distributed across meals.

Protein is not simply macronutrient math.

It is preservation strategy.

Resistance Training as Anti-Aging Medicine

Resistance training provides mechanical stimulus to muscle fibers. This stimulus activates signaling pathways that promote muscle maintenance and growth.

Without resistance stimulus:

Muscle mass declines

Strength decreases

Metabolic rate gradually lowers

Resistance training does not need to be extreme.

It requires:

Progressive overload

Consistency

Targeting major muscle groups

Recovery

Two to four sessions weekly can significantly influence long-term metabolic durability.

In aging populations, resistance training is not optional in weight management.

It is protective.

Women, Hormones, and Midlife Risk

For many women, midlife introduces additional metabolic variables:

Declining estrogen

Shifts in fat distribution

Reduced bone density

Increased visceral adiposity

Estrogen plays a role in fat distribution and insulin sensitivity. As levels decline, central adiposity often increases.

Rapid weight loss without muscle preservation during this phase may accelerate metabolic vulnerability.

For women over 35, muscle preservation becomes even more critical.

Weight reduction without resistance training may unintentionally compromise long-term stability.

Bone Density and Rapid Weight Loss

Bone remodeling is influenced by mechanical loading.

When body weight decreases significantly:

Mechanical stress on bone decreases

Bone density may decline if stimulus is insufficient

Resistance training mitigates this effect.

Adequate protein intake supports structural integrity.

Metabolic health includes skeletal health.

The Illusion of “Success”

Rapid scale reduction can create the appearance of improvement.

But if:

Lean mass declines

Strength decreases

Bone density weakens

Fat distribution shifts unfavorably

The long-term trajectory may be compromised.

Success must be defined by:

Composition

Strength

Stability

Function

Not simply numerical reduction.

The Aging-Aware Strategy

GLP-1 therapy can reduce appetite resistance.

It cannot override age-related muscle decline.

An aging-aware weight loss strategy includes:

Adequate protein intake

Structured resistance training

Sleep optimization

Stress regulation

Periodic reassessment

The objective is not minimal body weight.

It is preserved metabolic infrastructure across decades.

The Honest Perspective

Weight loss in youth is different from weight loss in midlife.

Biology shifts.

Resilience requires intention.

GLP-1 therapy may create opportunity.

Aging physiology demands structure.

Muscle is not aesthetic.

It is longevity.

Clinician Bottom Line GLP-1 therapy can reduce physiologic resistance to change, but it does not replace metabolic structure. The most durable outcomes occur when muscle preservation, nutritional strategy, realistic expectations, and clinical oversight remain central to the process. The goal is not simply rapid weight loss. The goal is long-term metabolic stability.

Chapter 8 - Safety, Monitoring, and Clinical Oversight

GLP-1 medications are powerful. Power requires oversight.

These therapies are generally well tolerated when appropriately prescribed. They are not cosmetic interventions. They are medical treatments.

Responsible use requires evaluation, monitoring, and structured follow-up.

Appropriate Evaluation

Before initiating therapy, a comprehensive medical review is essential.

This includes assessment of:

Endocrine history

Gastrointestinal history

Personal or family history of specific endocrine tumors

Current medications

Cardiometabolic risk profile

Treatment decisions should be individualized.

Standardized questionnaires cannot replace clinical reasoning.

Titration and Dose Adjustment

GLP-1 therapies are typically initiated at lower doses and titrated gradually.

This approach:

Improves tolerability

Allows physiologic adaptation

Escalating dose solely to accelerate weight loss is not evidence-based strategy.

Dose adjustments should reflect:

Clinical response

Tolerability

Metabolic indicators

Patient goals

Faster is not inherently safer or more effective.

Common Side Effects

The most frequently reported effects include:

Nausea

Early satiety

Gastrointestinal discomfort

Constipation or diarrhea

These symptoms often improve with gradual titration and dietary modification.

Persistent or severe symptoms require evaluation.

Education reduces unnecessary discontinuation.

Laboratory Monitoring

While not required universally, clinicians often monitor:

Hemoglobin A1c

Fasting glucose

Lipid profiles

Renal function

Hepatic markers when indicated

Monitoring reinforces that therapy is metabolic — not cosmetic.

Objective data informs clinical decisions.

When to Reevaluate

Therapy may need reassessment in cases of:

Intolerable side effects

Significant dehydration

Unexplained abdominal pain

Inadequate nutritional intake

Major life disruptions affecting stability

Medication should adapt to the patient — not the reverse.

Telehealth and Accountability

Expanded telehealth access has increased availability of treatment.

Access is beneficial. Access without structure is not.

Responsible prescribing includes:

Transparent risk discussion

Clear expectations

Defined follow-up intervals

Availability for questions

Long-term planning

Convenience must not eliminate clinical accountability.

Chronic Disease Framing

For some individuals, obesity represents a chronic metabolic condition. Long-term pharmacologic support may be appropriate.

For others, therapy may serve as a bridge.

Neither model is inherently superior.

The distinction lies in intention.

Treatment should exist within a defined plan — not as a short-term experiment.

Clinician Bottom Line GLP-1 therapy can reduce physiologic resistance to change, but it does not replace metabolic structure. The most durable outcomes occur when muscle preservation, nutritional strategy, realistic expectations, and clinical oversight remain central to the process. The goal is not simply rapid weight loss. The goal is long-term metabolic stability.

Chapter 9 - GLP-1 in Context: Other Medications and Interventions

No medication exists in isolation.

GLP-1 therapies represent a significant advancement in metabolic care. They are not the only option.

Clinical maturity is reflected not in enthusiasm for a single treatment – but in perspective.

Earlier Pharmacologic Options

Before GLP-1–based therapies became widely available, several medications were used for weight management, including:

Phentermine/topiramate

Bupropion/naltrexone

Orlistat

Metformin (in certain off-label contexts)

These agents operate through different mechanisms:

Central appetite stimulation or suppression

Reward pathway modulation

Reduced fat absorption

Improved insulin sensitivity

Effect sizes vary. Side-effect profiles differ. Some carry stimulant properties. Others require psychiatric or gastrointestinal caution.

No option is universally superior.

Selection depends on:

Clinical history

Risk profile

Tolerability

Treatment goals

Combination Therapy

In selected cases, combination pharmacotherapy may be considered.

This requires careful supervision.

Layering medications without structure increases risk. Thoughtful combination may enhance outcomes — but only when guided by clinical reasoning rather than urgency.

More medication is not inherently better medication.

Bariatric Surgery

Metabolic and bariatric surgery remains the most effective intervention for substantial and sustained weight reduction in appropriate candidates.

Surgical approaches:

Alter gastrointestinal anatomy

Influence hormonal signaling

Produce significant metabolic shifts

For individuals with severe obesity or significant comorbidities, surgery may achieve outcomes medication alone cannot replicate.

However, surgery carries procedural risk and requires lifelong nutritional monitoring.

GLP-1 therapy does not replace surgery. Surgery does not invalidate pharmacologic care.

Each occupies a distinct clinical space.

Lifestyle Intervention Alone

Nutritional structure, resistance training, sleep regulation, and stress management remain foundational regardless of pharmacologic support.

Some individuals achieve meaningful improvement through behavioral intervention alone. Others encounter persistent biological resistance despite structured effort.

Pharmacologic support does not eliminate behavioral responsibility. It may reduce physiologic resistance to it.

Chronic vs. Transitional Use

GLP-1 therapy may function within different models:

Short-term metabolic bridge

Medium-term support during restructuring

Long-term management of chronic obesity

There is no universal template.

Chronic conditions are often managed chronically.

Framing shapes expectation. Expectation shapes satisfaction.

The Balanced View

GLP-1 therapies are neither miracle cures nor last resorts.

They are clinical tools.

When integrated appropriately:

They can improve metabolic markers

They can reduce appetite resistance

They can support durable change

When treated as isolated solutions:

Expectations inflate

Structure weakens

Disappointment increases

Perspective protects outcomes. Context protects credibility.

The most responsible approach is rarely extreme.

It is structured.

Clinician Bottom Line GLP-1 therapy can reduce physiologic resistance to change, but it does not replace metabolic structure. The most durable outcomes occur when muscle preservation, nutritional strategy, realistic expectations, and clinical oversight remain central to the process. The goal is not simply rapid weight loss. The goal is long-term metabolic stability.

Chapter 10 - When GLP-1 Is the Right Tool — and When It's Not

GLP-1 medications are powerful. They are not universal.

Every responsible clinical decision begins with the same question:

Is this the right tool for this individual, at this time?

When It May Be Appropriate

For individuals living with:

Obesity

Insulin resistance

Type 2 diabetes

Elevated cardiometabolic risk

Repeated weight regain despite structured effort

GLP-1 therapy may provide meaningful metabolic support.

Potential improvements include:

Reduced appetite resistance

Improved glycemic control

Lower blood pressure

Favorable lipid changes

Reduced visceral adiposity

In these contexts, the objective is not cosmetic change. It is metabolic stabilization.

When Structural Drivers Dominate

Not all weight challenges originate from the same mechanisms.

Some individuals are primarily navigating:

Chronic sleep deprivation

Persistent stress

Untreated mood disorders

Medication-induced weight changes

Disordered eating patterns

Inconsistent nutritional structure

In these situations, appetite suppression alone may produce temporary reduction without resolving underlying drivers.

Medication does not replace sleep. It does not resolve chronic stress. It does not treat disordered eating.

In such cases, behavioral or psychological intervention may be primary.

Aesthetic-Driven Use

Another category warrants careful discussion: individuals seeking modest aesthetic refinement despite stable metabolic health.

When the primary objective is cosmetic rather than medical, the risk–benefit discussion shifts.

Weight reduction for metabolic protection and weight reduction for aesthetic preference are not identical conversations.

Intent matters.

Contraindications and Caution

Certain medical histories require caution or avoidance, including:

Specific endocrine tumor histories

Certain gastrointestinal conditions

Significant malnutrition risk

Tolerability concerns

Clinical screening protects safety.

Eligibility is not about worth. It is about suitability.

Engagement and Durability

Even in appropriate candidates, outcomes depend on engagement.

If an individual is unwilling to:

Prioritize protein intake

Incorporate resistance training

Stabilize sleep

Participate in monitoring

Medication becomes the entire strategy.

Entire strategies rarely endure.

When GLP-1 therapy is used as a metabolic bridge — reducing physiologic resistance while structural habits are built — long-term durability improves.

The molecule does not determine success. The model does.

Clear Criteria

GLP-1 therapy is most appropriate when:

Metabolic dysfunction is present

Appetite dysregulation is significant

Structural reinforcement is planned

Monitoring is ongoing

Expectations are realistic

It is less appropriate when:

The goal is rapid cosmetic change

Foundational behaviors are absent

Oversight is minimal

Education is superficial

GLP-1 therapy is neither miracle nor moral compromise.

It is a clinical tool.

Applied thoughtfully, it alters trajectories. Applied casually, it alters numbers.

Clinician Bottom Line GLP-1 therapy can reduce physiologic resistance to change, but it does not replace metabolic structure. The most durable outcomes occur when muscle preservation, nutritional strategy, realistic expectations, and clinical oversight remain central to the process. The goal is not simply rapid weight loss. The goal is long-term metabolic stability.

Chapter 11 - Coming Off the Medication: The Truth

Most conversations about GLP-1 therapy focus on how to begin.

Fewer address how — or whether — to stop.

Eventually, the question emerges:

"How long will I need to stay on this?"

The honest answer is individualized. There is no universal endpoint.

What Happens Biologically

GLP-1 medications modulate appetite signaling and metabolic regulation while active in the system.

When discontinued, those signals gradually return toward baseline.

This is not failure. It is pharmacology.

If medication has been performing most of the regulatory work — suppressing appetite without structural reinforcement — hunger may feel amplified when it returns.

If medication has been used as a metabolic bridge — supporting protein prioritization, resistance training, and behavioral stabilization — outcomes are often more durable.

The difference is preparation.

What the Evidence Suggests

Clinical data show that some individuals experience partial or significant weight regain after discontinuation.

This should not create fear. It should create planning.

Chronic metabolic dysregulation does not resolve permanently after short-term modulation.

Weight regulation remains biologically defended.

Expectation shapes interpretation.

Chronic Disease Framing

For many individuals, obesity is a chronic condition.

Long-term pharmacologic support may be appropriate — just as it is in hypertension, dyslipidemia, or diabetes management.

Remaining on medication is not dependency. It may be management.

Discontinuation is not moral superiority. It is a clinical decision.

Neutral framing removes stigma.

Preparing for Transition

If therapy is reduced or discontinued, structure becomes more important — not less.

Preparation may include:

Maintaining adequate protein intake

Preserving resistance training

Anticipating normalized hunger signals

Reinforcing meal consistency

Monitoring metabolic markers

Hunger returning is not failure. It is physiology.

Without preparation, appetite resurgence may feel destabilizing. With preparation, it feels predictable.

The Psychological Narrative

Discontinuation can trigger internal narratives:

“I should be able to maintain this alone.” “If I regain, I failed.”

These narratives oversimplify chronic biology.

Medication assists regulation. Structure determines durability.

No medication permanently erases metabolic defense mechanisms.

Understanding this before initiation changes how discontinuation feels later.

The Honest Framing

GLP-1 therapy is not a temporary trick. It is not a guaranteed permanent reset.

It is a metabolic tool.

Duration depends on:

Individual physiology

Comorbidity burden

Risk tolerance

Structural reinforcement

Clinical goals

The injection may stop.

The system should not.

Clinician Bottom Line GLP-1 therapy can reduce physiologic resistance to change, but it does not replace metabolic structure. The most durable outcomes occur when muscle preservation, nutritional strategy, realistic expectations, and clinical oversight remain central to the process. The goal is not simply rapid weight loss. The goal is long-term metabolic stability.

Chapter 12 - Constructing Metabolic Infrastructure

Weight loss is an event. Metabolic resilience is a system.

GLP-1 therapy can create momentum. Appetite quiets. Portions decrease. The scale reflects measurable change.

Momentum is temporary. Infrastructure determines permanence.

Protein as Structural Priority

When appetite declines, intake often declines with it.

Without intention, protein consumption may fall below levels necessary to preserve lean mass.

Muscle maintenance requires adequate amino acid availability. During weight reduction, protein must be deliberate — not incidental.

Protein becomes structural. Not optional.

Resistance Training as Metabolic Insurance

Skeletal muscle is metabolically active tissue. It supports:

Insulin sensitivity

Glucose disposal

Resting energy expenditure

Functional independence

Without resistance stimulus, muscle declines during caloric reduction.

Strength training does not need to be extreme. It needs to be consistent.

Two to four weekly sessions targeting major muscle groups can significantly influence long-term metabolic durability.

The objective is preservation. Not performance.

Daily Movement and Energy Output

Non-exercise activity thermogenesis (NEAT) — daily movement outside structured workouts — contributes meaningfully to total energy expenditure.

Walking, standing, occupational activity, and household movement all matter.

When weight decreases, spontaneous movement may decline unconsciously.

Structured exercise is important. Daily movement sustains baseline metabolic output.

Sleep and Hormonal Stability

Chronic sleep restriction disrupts:

Ghrelin (hunger signaling)

Leptin (satiety signaling)

Cortisol (stress hormone)

Glucose tolerance

No medication overrides persistent sleep deprivation.

Seven to eight hours of restorative sleep is not optional in metabolic care.

It is infrastructure.

Stress Regulation

Chronic stress influences appetite, food preference, insulin sensitivity, and fat distribution.

Elevated cortisol contributes to visceral adiposity and metabolic instability.

Stress management is physiologic regulation — not lifestyle luxury.

Structured recovery, boundaries, and nervous system regulation directly affect metabolic durability.

Nutritional Structure Beyond Calories

GLP-1 therapy reduces hunger. It does not define nutritional quality.

Lower intake does not guarantee adequate micronutrients.

Intentional meal composition — sufficient protein, fiber, minimally processed foods — supports energy stability and recovery.

Medication suppresses appetite. Structure defines nourishment.

Redefining Success

Infrastructure reframes success.

Not solely:

Pounds lost

Clothing size

But also:

Strength preserved

Energy stable

Laboratory markers improved

Appetite predictable

Stress regulated

The objective is not minimal body weight.

It is maximal metabolic resilience.

Clinician Bottom Line GLP-1 therapy can reduce physiologic resistance to change, but it does not replace metabolic structure. The most durable outcomes occur when muscle preservation, nutritional strategy, realistic expectations, and clinical oversight remain central to the process. The goal is not simply rapid weight loss. The goal is long-term metabolic stability.

Chapter 13 - What Actually Matters

GLP-1 medications have changed the weight conversation.

They have increased access. They have reduced stigma for some. They have introduced confusion for others.

The medication itself is not the controversy.

The misunderstanding is.

In clinical practice, the most common challenge is not whether GLP-1 therapy works. It often does. The deeper challenge is how quickly the conversation shifts away from physiology and toward expectation. Rapid results create urgency. Visibility creates comparison. And comparison rarely produces durable strategy.

What ultimately determines long-term outcomes is not the molecule alone. It is the model surrounding it.

The Tool vs. The Model

GLP-1 therapy can:

• Reduce appetite resistance • Improve glycemic control • Support meaningful weight reduction • Improve select cardiometabolic markers

For many individuals, this is the first experience of biological alignment rather than constant resistance.

But medication is not a model. It is a tool within a larger system.

Used thoughtfully, it becomes leverage. Used in isolation, it becomes temporary.

A quieter appetite does not automatically create structure. Without reinforcement—protein sufficiency, resistance training, sleep stability, and realistic expectations—the early momentum fades and frustration returns.

The injection influences signaling. Structure determines permanence.

Weight Loss vs. Metabolic Durability

Weight loss is visible. Metabolic durability is structural.

Durability includes:

• Preserved lean mass • Stable glucose regulation • Sustainable energy patterns • Psychological alignment • Behavioral reinforcement

A lower number on the scale does not guarantee resilience. Rapid reduction does not guarantee maintenance. Silence of appetite does not equal restored physiology.

The body adapts. Always.

Durable outcomes occur when the period of reduced appetite is used to strengthen the metabolic foundation—not simply accelerate reduction.

Neutral Framing Removes Shame

GLP-1 therapy is not a moral decision. It is a clinical one.

Remaining on medication long term may be appropriate. Transitioning off may also be appropriate.

Neither reflects discipline. Neither reflects failure.

Obesity and metabolic dysregulation exist on a spectrum influenced by biology, environment, and behavior. Framing treatment choices through morality creates unnecessary stigma and unrealistic expectations.

Biology is not ideology.

When neutrality replaces judgment, decision-making becomes clearer and more sustainable.

Clarity Over Extremes

Public narratives tend toward extremes:

Miracle. Shortcut. Cheating. Cure.

Extremes simplify complex physiology into slogans.

Clinical reality is quieter.

GLP-1 therapies represent a meaningful advancement in metabolic care. They reduce friction within systems that were previously resistant to change. But they do not eliminate the need for:

• Nutritional structure • Muscle preservation • Sleep regulation • Stress management • Ongoing oversight

Medication can initiate change. Structure sustains it.

The Real Objective

The goal of metabolic care is not minimal body weight.

It is maximal physiologic stability.

It is the ability to maintain energy without constant negotiation. To preserve muscle while reducing adiposity. To move through daily life without persistent metabolic friction.

The most durable outcomes are rarely the most dramatic. They are the most structured.

GLP-1 therapy can create opportunity.

Opportunity requires intention. Intention builds structure. Structure builds resilience.

The Honest Perspective

This book was not written to promote a trend. It was written to restore context.

GLP-1 medications are neither miracle solutions nor moral compromises. They are biologic tools—effective when applied thoughtfully, disappointing when treated as complete solutions.

What actually matters is not the speed of change. It is the stability that follows it.

What actually matters is not the injection itself. It is the system built around it.

And ultimately, what actually matters is not simply losing weight.

It is building a body—and a metabolic environment—that can sustain health long after the initial momentum slows.

— Sylvalene Alozie, DNP, APRN, FNP-C

Clinician Bottom Line GLP-1 therapy can reduce physiologic resistance to change, but it does not replace metabolic structure. The most durable outcomes occur when muscle preservation, nutritional strategy, realistic expectations, and clinical oversight remain central to the process. The goal is not simply rapid weight loss. The goal is long-term metabolic stability.

Chapter 14 - Long-Term Maintenance Models

Weight loss is common. Maintenance is rare.

GLP-1 therapy has altered how weight is reduced. It has not eliminated the biology that defends regain.

Long-term outcomes depend less on how weight is lost and more on how maintenance is structured.

There is no single model that applies to everyone.

But there are recognizable patterns.

Model 1: Chronic Pharmacologic Support

For some individuals, obesity functions as a chronic metabolic condition.

In these cases:

Appetite dysregulation is persistent

Insulin resistance is significant

Weight regain follows every prior intervention

For these individuals, long-term pharmacologic support may be appropriate.

This model mirrors other chronic disease frameworks:

Antihypertensives for blood pressure

Statins for dyslipidemia

Insulin for diabetes

Remaining on medication long term is not dependency.

It may be management.

The goal in this model is stability — not cycling.

Structure remains essential:

Protein sufficiency

Resistance training

Periodic monitoring

Dose reassessment over time

Medication assists regulation. Behavior sustains function.

Model 2: Metabolic Bridge

Some individuals use GLP-1 therapy as a temporary metabolic bridge.

In this model:

Appetite resistance is reduced

Weight decreases

Structural habits are built

Muscle is preserved

Sleep and stress are stabilized

After sufficient reinforcement, medication may be tapered.

This model requires preparation.

Without structural reinforcement, bridge models collapse.

With structure, they may succeed.

The critical variable is not duration.

It is foundation.

Model 3: Cyclical Support

A third pattern involves intermittent or cyclical use under supervision.

In this model:

Medication is used during high-risk periods

Reinforcement strategies are revisited

Maintenance phases alternate with short support periods

This approach requires clinical oversight.

Unsupervised cycling may destabilize appetite signaling and expectation.

Cyclical support is strategic — not reactive.

Model 4: Integrated Surgical + Pharmacologic Care

In individuals who undergo bariatric surgery, GLP-1 therapy may later be used to support weight stability or manage regain.

Surgery alters anatomy and hormonal signaling. Medication may complement those changes.

These approaches are not competitive.

They are layered.

Integrated care often produces durable outcomes when structure remains intact.

Why Maintenance Fails

Maintenance failure often reflects one or more of the following:

Lean mass loss during weight reduction

Unrealistic expectations

Absence of resistance training

Nutritional structure erosion

Psychological fatigue

Belief that medication alone determines permanence

The body defends equilibrium.

If structure weakens while appetite returns, regain becomes biologically probable.

This is not moral failure.

It is physiologic predictability.

The Maintenance Mindset Shift

Early weight loss rewards urgency.

Maintenance rewards maturity.

The shift includes:

From speed to sustainability From restriction to structure From scale obsession to metabolic metrics From temporary strategy to system

This psychological transition is often more difficult than the initial loss phase.

But it determines durability.

The Honest Truth

There is no universally "correct" duration for GLP-1 therapy.

There is only appropriate context.

The key questions are:

What biology am I managing?

What structure have I built?

What is my long-term risk profile?

What model aligns with my physiology?

Medication may be long term. It may be transitional. It may be supportive.

But it is never the entire system.

The Durable Framework

Sustainable maintenance requires:

Preserved muscle mass

Adequate protein intake

Resistance training

Stable sleep

Stress regulation

Periodic clinical reassessment

Realistic expectation

GLP-1 therapy may reduce friction.

Structure determines permanence.

Chapter 15 - Clinical Monitoring and Metabolic Oversight

GLP-1 therapy is not cosmetic care.

It is metabolic intervention.

Any intervention that alters appetite, insulin signaling, and body composition warrants structured oversight.

Responsible prescribing includes monitoring — not simply dispensing.

Baseline Assessment

Before initiating therapy, a structured baseline evaluation establishes context.

This may include:

Weight and body composition (when available)

Blood pressure

Hemoglobin A1c

Fasting glucose

Lipid profile

Liver function markers

Renal function

Not every patient requires every test.

But baseline data clarifies trajectory.

Weight reduction without metabolic context is incomplete.

Ongoing Laboratory Monitoring

During therapy, periodic reassessment may be appropriate depending on clinical context.

Common markers include:

Hemoglobin A1c

Fasting glucose

Lipid profile

Renal function

Hepatic markers

In individuals with diabetes or prediabetes, glucose monitoring may be more frequent.

Objective data informs adjustment.

Monitoring reinforces that therapy is metabolic — not aesthetic.

Nutritional Surveillance

Reduced appetite can unintentionally lead to inadequate intake.

Monitoring includes attention to:

Protein sufficiency

Hydration status

Micronutrient adequacy

Gastrointestinal tolerance

Persistent nausea, dehydration, or prolonged low intake warrants reassessment.

Appetite reduction is therapeutic. Malnutrition is not.

Hydration and Electrolytes

Delayed gastric emptying and reduced intake may affect hydration patterns.

Encouraging:

Adequate fluid intake

Electrolyte balance

Gradual titration

reduces preventable side effects.

Dizziness, persistent fatigue, or orthostatic symptoms should not be ignored.

Gastrointestinal Adaptation

Nausea and satiety changes are common during dose escalation.

Gradual titration reduces severity.

Dietary adjustments — smaller meals, adequate protein, slower eating — often improve tolerability.

Persistent abdominal pain requires evaluation.

Symptoms should be assessed, not dismissed.

Body Composition Awareness

While not mandatory in all settings, awareness of body composition enhances clinical insight.

If available, periodic evaluation of lean mass and fat mass distribution can inform strategy.

Strength metrics may serve as functional indicators of preservation.

Weight alone does not define progress.

When to Reevaluate Therapy

Therapy should be reassessed when:

Side effects are intolerable

Nutritional intake becomes inadequate

Psychological distress increases

Life circumstances destabilize routine

Goals shift

Medication should serve the patient.

Not the reverse.

The Telehealth Responsibility

Expanded access through telehealth increases availability.

Availability does not eliminate accountability.

Responsible virtual prescribing includes:

Structured intake

Clear education

Defined follow-up intervals

Accessible communication

Documented risk discussion

Convenience must not replace oversight.

Chronic Care Framing

If obesity is chronic, monitoring should be longitudinal.

Chronic conditions require periodic reassessment — not episodic intervention.

Stability is maintained through review, adjustment, and reinforcement.

The objective is not indefinite escalation.

It is appropriate alignment.

The Clinical Standard

GLP-1 therapy can be powerful.

Power demands structure.

Monitoring is not fear-based.

It is responsible care.

It protects the patient. It protects the clinician. It protects the outcome.

Medication may reduce appetite.

Oversight protects physiology.

Chapter 16 - Case-Based Clinical Scenarios

Metabolic care is not theoretical.

It unfolds in real time — across different physiologies, expectations, and life contexts.

The following composite cases illustrate common patterns observed during GLP-1 therapy.

Case 1: The Rapid Responder

Profile: Female, 38, insulin resistance, prior dieting history, high occupational stress.

Within the first 12 weeks of therapy:

Appetite decreased substantially

Weight reduced rapidly

Food preoccupation diminished

Energy improved

Early success created optimism.

However, protein intake declined unintentionally. Resistance training remained inconsistent.

At four months:

Strength decreased

Fatigue increased

Weight loss slowed

Intervention focused on:

Protein prioritization

Structured resistance training

Sleep stabilization

Weight loss continued more gradually. Strength improved.

Lesson: Rapid responders still require structure. Speed without reinforcement compromises durability.

Case 2: The Slow Responder

Profile: Male, 52, prediabetes, visceral adiposity, prior weight cycling.

After three months:

Modest scale reduction

Improved glycemic markers

Reduced hunger intensity

The patient expressed frustration: “It’s not working fast enough.”

However:

Fasting glucose improved

Waist circumference decreased

Energy stability increased

Expectation recalibration was necessary.

Weight reduction accelerated gradually over time as structure improved.

Lesson: Scale velocity does not equal metabolic success. Slow responders often demonstrate strong metabolic improvement before visible change.

Case 3: The Plateau Phase

Profile: Female, 45, perimenopausal, high baseline stress.

Initial loss was steady. At month five, progress stalled.

Evaluation revealed:

Reduced resistance training

Increased occupational stress

Inconsistent sleep

Gradual protein decline

No immediate dose escalation occurred.

Intervention prioritized:

Sleep normalization

Stress reduction

Recommitment to strength training

Weight loss resumed gradually.

Lesson: Plateaus often reflect structural drift – not medication failure.

Case 4: Discontinuation Without Preparation

Profile: Male, 41, no prior strength training history.

Weight reduction was significant over six months.

The patient discontinued medication abruptly due to cost concerns.

Within three months:

Appetite increased sharply

Food preoccupation returned

Resistance training remained absent

Weight regain began

The patient interpreted regain as personal failure.

Reframing and structural reinforcement were required before reintroducing therapy.

Lesson: Discontinuation without preparation amplifies biological defense mechanisms.

Case 5: Long-Term Management Model

Profile: Female, 56, type 2 diabetes, long-standing obesity.

After structured weight reduction:

Glycemic control improved

Blood pressure decreased

Lean mass preserved through consistent strength training

Given chronic metabolic profile, long-term pharmacologic support was chosen.

Dose adjustments were made gradually. Monitoring continued.

Weight stabilized. Metabolic markers remained improved.

Lesson: For some individuals, chronic pharmacologic management is appropriate and stabilizing.

Case 6: Aesthetic-Driven Use

Profile: Female, 29, BMI at lower treatment threshold, primary motivation cosmetic.

Early weight loss occurred.

However:

Minimal resistance training

Irregular eating patterns

Psychological preoccupation with body image

Progress slowed. Anxiety increased.

After evaluation, therapy was discontinued. Behavioral support became primary.

Lesson: When structural and psychological drivers dominate, medication alone does not resolve instability.

Patterns Across Cases

Despite differences in physiology and trajectory, several themes recur:

Muscle preservation predicts durability

Sleep disruption predicts instability

Expectation misalignment predicts dissatisfaction

Abrupt discontinuation predicts regain

Structure predicts sustainability

Medication modulates signaling.

Behavior determines trajectory.

The Clinical Perspective

GLP-1 therapy is not a uniform experience.

Some individuals lose weight rapidly. Some gradually. Some plateau early. Some maintain long term.

Outcomes reflect:

Baseline physiology

Structural reinforcement

Psychological alignment

Monitoring consistency

The objective is not identical results.

It is appropriate alignment.

Chapter 17 - Clinical Myths and GLP-1 Misinterpretations

GLP-1 therapy exists in a climate of amplified opinion.

Public conversation often polarizes quickly.

Miracle. Shortcut. Cheating. Dangerous. Cure.

Extremes simplify complex biology.

Clarity requires nuance.

Myth 1: “It’s Just an Easy Way Out”

This assumption rests on the belief that weight regulation is purely behavioral.

It is not.

Appetite signaling, insulin sensitivity, reward circuitry, and metabolic adaptation influence weight regulation independent of intention.

GLP-1 therapy reduces physiologic resistance.

It does not remove responsibility.

Medication may lower the barrier.

Structure still determines outcome.

Myth 2: “Once You Start, You’re on It Forever”

There is no universal rule.

Some individuals use therapy as a metabolic bridge. Others require long-term support.

Chronic diseases are often managed chronically.

Hypertension is not “cured” with short-term treatment. Neither is insulin resistance.

Duration depends on physiology – not ideology.

Myth 3: “You’ll Regain Everything Immediately”

Regain risk varies.

If lean mass is preserved and structure reinforced, maintenance may be stable.

If appetite suppression was the only strategy, regain becomes more likely.

The medication does not determine permanence.

Preparation does.

Myth 4: “It Destroys Metabolism”

GLP-1 therapy does not inherently damage metabolic function.

However, rapid weight loss without muscle preservation may lower resting metabolic rate.

The difference lies in strategy.

Muscle preservation protects metabolic capacity.

Aggressive caloric restriction without structure weakens it.

Myth 5: “It Works the Same for Everyone”

Response variability is normal.

Factors influencing outcomes include:

Baseline insulin resistance

Visceral adiposity

Age

Sleep patterns

Stress load

Lean mass preservation

Genetic predisposition

Some individuals lose rapidly. Others gradually. Some plateau early.

Variation is physiology — not failure.

Myth 6: “It’s Purely Cosmetic”

While some pursue therapy for aesthetic reasons, GLP-1 medications were developed for metabolic disease.

Clinical trials demonstrate improvements in:

Glycemic control

Cardiovascular risk markers

Weight-related comorbidities

The medication is not inherently cosmetic.

The context determines the objective.

Myth 7: “It Replaces Lifestyle”

No medication replaces sleep.

No injection builds muscle.

No prescription stabilizes stress.

GLP-1 therapy may reduce appetite resistance.

It does not eliminate the need for:

Protein sufficiency

Resistance training

Sleep hygiene

Stress regulation

When treated as a substitute, it disappoints.

When treated as support, it stabilizes.

Myth 8: “It’s Unsafe by Default”

All medications carry risk.

Risk must be contextualized.

When prescribed appropriately, titrated gradually, and monitored responsibly, GLP-1 therapies are generally well tolerated.

Safety is not determined by headlines.

It is determined by screening, supervision, and structure.

Myth 9: “Weight Loss Equals Health”

Weight reduction may improve health markers.

It does not automatically guarantee metabolic resilience.

Preserved muscle, stable glucose regulation, sleep quality, and stress control matter.

The objective is not minimal mass.

It is physiologic stability.

The Larger Misinterpretation

The most persistent misconception is that GLP-1 therapy is either a miracle or a moral compromise.

It is neither.

It is a tool.

Tools are neither virtuous nor flawed.

They are effective when applied appropriately.

The Neutral Position

Clinical maturity resists extremes.

GLP-1 therapy:

Is not magic

Is not cheating

Is not universally necessary

Is not universally inappropriate

It is a biologic intervention within a broader metabolic model.

Clarity stabilizes decision-making.

Extremes distort it.

Appendix

The GLP-1 Readiness Checklist

Before initiating GLP-1 therapy, pause.

This is not a test.

It is preparation.

Clarity before initiation improves outcomes after initiation.

1. Medical Readiness

Have I reviewed my complete medical history with a qualified healthcare professional? Do I understand the potential side effects and expected tolerability profile? Have appropriate laboratory assessments been discussed, if clinically indicated? Do I understand realistic average weight-loss expectations — not social media outcomes?

2. Expectation Clarity

Am I prepared for weight loss to slow over time? Do I understand that plateau phases are physiologic, not failure? Do I accept that the scale is one metric — not the sole measure of progress? Am I prepared for appetite signals to return if the medication is discontinued?

3. Nutritional Structure

Do I have a clear plan to prioritize adequate protein intake? Am I prepared to eat intentionally, even when hunger is reduced? Do I understand the risk of lean mass loss during rapid weight reduction?

4. Movement and Muscle

Am I willing to incorporate consistent resistance training? Do I understand that muscle preservation supports metabolic durability? Am I prepared to prioritize strength, not just weight?

5. Long-Term Perspective

Have I considered whether this treatment is short-term, transitional, or long-term? Do I understand that medication is a tool — not the entire strategy? Am I committed to building structural habits while appetite resistance is reduced?

Final Reflection

If most responses are yes, GLP-1 therapy may function as a powerful metabolic bridge.

If many responses are no, pause.

Preparation strengthens durability.

Medication may reduce appetite.

Only structure builds sustainability.

Who This Book Is For

This guide is written for individuals who are considering GLP-1 therapy, currently using it, or seeking a clearer understanding of how weight-loss medications fit within long-term metabolic health.

It is for those who want context beyond headlines.

It is for those who prefer physiology over hype.

It is for those who understand that sustainable change requires structure.

This book is also relevant for clinicians who want a balanced, behaviorally informed framework for discussing GLP-1 therapy with patients.

The purpose of this guide is not to promote treatment.

It is not to discourage treatment.

It is to clarify it.

Clarity improves decisions.

And informed decisions improve outcomes.

ABOUT THE AUTHOR

Sylvalene Alozie, DNP, APRN, FNP-C is a doctoral-prepared nurse practitioner specializing in metabolic health and evidence-based weight management. She provides virtual clinical consultations for adults seeking structured, medically grounded guidance in GLP-1 therapy and long-term metabolic care.

Her clinical approach emphasizes individualized assessment, thoughtful medication use, muscle preservation, and behavioral reinforcement — what she describes as a structure-first model of metabolic treatment. She believes that sustainable results are built through clarity, physiology, and consistency rather than urgency or trends.

In both practice and writing, Dr. Alozie is committed to reducing confusion around weight-loss therapy and helping patients make informed, balanced decisions about their health.

NOTES

www.ingramcontent.com/pod-product-compliance
Lightning Source LLC
LaVergne TN
LVHW050939210926
848482LV00013B/667
* 9 7 9 8 2 9 5 6 6 5 7 2 1 *